Reina Carolina Vargas Argote

Acne:

Reina Carolina Vargas Argote

# Acne:

## Aetiology, Pathophysiology, Typologies and Treatments

ScienciaScripts

**Imprint**

Any brand names and product names mentioned in this book are subject to trademark, brand or patent protection and are trademarks or registered trademarks of their respective holders. The use of brand names, product names, common names, trade names, product descriptions etc. even without a particular marking in this work is in no way to be construed to mean that such names may be regarded as unrestricted in respect of trademark and brand protection legislation and could thus be used by anyone.

Cover image: www.ingimage.com

This book is a translation from the original published under ISBN 978-620-2-25485-4.

Publisher:
Sciencia Scripts
is a trademark of
International Book Market Service Ltd., member of OmniScriptum Publishing Group
17 Meldrum Street, Beau Bassin 71504, Mauritius
Printed at: see last page
**ISBN: 978-620-3-48254-6**

**Title:**

*Acne: Etiology, Pathophysiology, Typologies and Treatments*


**Author:**

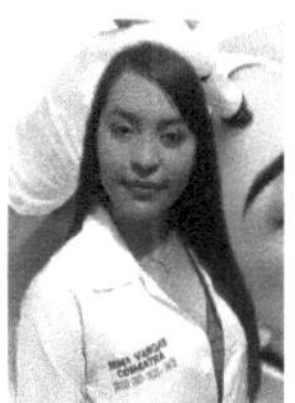

### *Reina Carolina Vargas Argote*

*Cosmiatrist*
*Specialist in Cosmiátricos Acids Speaker Medium Technician in Electromedicine and Pharmaceutical Independent Researcher - Venezuela*
*ORCID: https://orcid.org/0000-0003-3872-7304 E-mail: reinadevalera123@gmail.com*


## Methodological Reviewer:

### *MSc. Betty De La Hoz Suarez*

*Accredited Researcher and Scientific Articulist Reviewer and International Referee Member of the Scientific Committee of Refereed and Editorial Journals Editor-in-Chief of the Journal Innovación Estética.*
*Member Center: INDECSAR Group - Ecuador ORCID: https://orcid.org/0000-0002-5800-9775*
*E-mail: editorial@indecsar.org*

# Table of Contents

# FOREWORD

Medicine, seen from a scientific point of view, is in constant and continuous change. Every day new medical discoveries are made, new causes of diseases are found, advanced and novel treatments are experimented, new therapeutic techniques are discovered, more preventive treatments come to light, and, as if that were not enough, the ways of making pathological diagnoses are changed. It is precisely research and clinical experience that allow knowledge to be expanded and these discoveries and advances in medicine to be made known.

Research on the etiology of acne has progressed tremendously in recent years. Studies of acne pathology from the perspectives of sebaceous glands, sebum production, keratinization, differentiation, bacterial proliferation, genetics, immunology, wound healing, among others, have gradually clarified its pathogenesis. This has led to the development of new treatments, therapies and techniques, which are paving the way for important and profound studies that will allow a better evolution of acne treatment.

Acne represents one of the most frequent reasons for dermatological consultation in all types of people, but especially in adolescents, and, as a multifactorial disease observable in the skin, it must be attended and treated in an adequate and effective manner, making it essential and strictly necessary to know its causes or origin. With this in mind, the present work has as its initial objective to analyze the pathogenesis or etiology of acne, as well as its typologies and physiopathologies.

Acne, as one of the most common skin diseases, has been studied by a variety of dermatological specialists, during different decades, in order to find the most appropriate treatment to combat it. However, the etiology or pathogenesis of acne has led to the discovery that there is no single treatment to control or combat this disease. Therefore, the present work also analyzes the different types of treatments used to treat acne, according to its etiology and diagnosis.

The book consists of four chapters, the first one entitled *"Acne: Etiology and Definition"*, shows the origin, pathogenesis or the causes of acne as a dermatological disease; from the medical etiology, ancient and current. Once the etiological aspects of acne have been established, a series of definitions of the term are presented, from the point of view of various researchers and from the conception of the author of this work.The second chapter entitled *"Acne: Pathophysiology"*, studies the physical characteristics or functional changes associated with acne. Pathophysiology studies all those mechanisms of disease creation at the molecular, subcellular, cellular, tissue, organic and anatomical levels. The third chapter, entitled *"Acne: Typologies"*, shows the different types of acne based on various theoretical postulates. To speak of typologies is to know the types or models used to classify something. Typology is considered a science that studies the kinds or types of a matter in question; or the conceptual and intuitive difference of things. It is commonly used in terms of systematic studies in different areas with the purpose of defining categories. In this particular case, it is intended to classify acne with a specific focus on its different manifestations, symptoms and degrees.

The fourth chapter is entitled *"Acne: Treatments"*, and analyzes the different types of treatments used to treat acne, according to its etiology and diagnosis. The study focuses on treatments of different types, such as hormonal, systemic, topical and therapeutic, based on specialized, complex or even simple applications, which have already been proven to cure or control acne.

Considering the content of the book, there is no doubt that we are in the presence of a whole compendium of therapeutic possibilities and complementary and associative treatments, which not only remain in the common and widely used topical protocols and systemic therapies, but goes beyond, for example, procedures in which drugs are combined with physical methods, such as photoluminescent therapy. As an important feature, before choosing a treatment, the book places special emphasis on the pathogenesis, clinical type of acne, intensity, severity, skin phototype, depth, and even the degree of collaboration of the patient suffering from the disease.

With all certainty, the book *"Acne: Etiology, Physiopathology, Typology and Treatments"*, will be a research guide not only for health professionals, such as: Dermatologists, Dermocosmiatrists, Cosmiatrists, Cosmetologists, among others, but also for practical experts in the management of acne, students of Health Sciences, Aesthetics and Beauty in general, as well as, people of society who suffer from the disease; who, in one way or another, wish to be nourished about the pathogenesis of their acne, and the different treatment alternatives that exist to successfully treat the disease.

I hope that the work can awaken a special interest in the reader, and that its content can be used in the best possible way; that it can be a further contribution to scientific knowledge, and an additional door to the realization of new researches. I leave open the possibility for the reader to make his own decisions when choosing a treatment for acne, especially when it comes to dosages or specific applications. When in doubt, never fail to consult your physician.


*Reina Carolina Vargas Argote*

## DEDICATION

I dedicate this book first and foremost to Jehovah God, who has showered me with blessings to be able to carry out this intellectual project. With his help, power and encouragement, I was able to understand the words of Proverbs 10:22 "The blessings of the LORD are what enriches".

Secondly, to my husband and son who have been by my side all this time, giving me their support and sharing together the desire and desire to make this book possible. This achievement is also yours.

I also dedicate it to all those family members who are far away, but whom I love with all my heart. In particular, to Piedad Argote, my mother, who, with her love and words of encouragement, has always advised me not to give up, even in the midst of difficult circumstances.

I also dedicate it to Dilia, more than a friend, an advisor. One of those friends who doesn't let you fall, and if you fall, she picks you up.

Finally, to my dear Ospino friends, whose support was a fundamental part of this achievement.

*Reina Carolina Vargas Argote*

# INTRODUCTION

Acne is a skin disease that occurs when hair follicles become clogged. It is a chronic inflammation of the pilosebaceous follicles of the face, neck, thorax, arms and back; and it is more frequent in males during adolescence and in females in adulthood. According to the Chilean Society of Dermatology and Venerology, it affects between 70% and 85% of the general population worldwide.

Acne has been considered one of the most frequent dermatological pathologies, affecting almost 80% of adolescents between 13 and 18 years of age. Statisticians indicate that, of the number of dermatological consultations of adult patients, approximately 25% are due to acne. In the vast majority of cases, it can last for many years, leave physical and emotional sequelae and cause significant adverse effects on the psychological development of adolescents in society. (Grimalt, n/d).

Following this same order of ideas, White (1998), adds another interesting fact, and that is that acne usually occurs at puberty with a peak prevalence of 85% between the ages of 12 to 24 years. It should be noted, according to Ruiz (2018), that before 1980 acne was considered a problem only of adolescence, but gradually people of adult age were included. Today, it has been proven that acne also affects a large group of adult women, from 14% to more than 50%.

In addition, in people over the age of 25 years, the presence of acne is recorded at 3% in men and 12% in women; this percentage decreases in patients over 45 years of age, which can be as low as 1%. In most cases, acne may disappear in early adulthood, however, there are important sequelae reflected in the form of physical and psychological scars, which make the healing process of the disease longer (Goulden, Stables, & Cunliffe, 1999; Nast, Dreno, Bettoli, & Degitz, 2012).

On the other hand, there is a diversity of factors that can cause acne, among which can be mentioned excessive oil production, obstruction of the hair follicles with oil and dead cells, presence of bacteria, excess activity of a type of hormone, bad eating habits; however, these can be joined by many more, such as hereditary factors. In studies that have been carried out in this regard, it was shown that almost 20% of cases with moderate and severe acne have a family history. (Ghodsi, Orawa, & Zouboulis, 2009)

The severity of acne is established based on its extension, and will depend on the number of areas involved with the disease, as well as its percentage of affection. In this regard, it can be said that approximately 80% of patients with acne present mild disease and 14% moderate to severe. On the other hand, scars are present in 1% to 12% of patients who have been treated for acne. (Nast, Dreno, Bettoli, & Degitz, 2012).

On the other hand, knowledge about acne as a dermatological disease and its treatments has evolved favorably, which has generated controversies that have helped to eliminate beliefs, remove uncertainties, discover new techniques and face realities. As research on the subject continues, new doubts arise, from which new truths and new advances in its etiology and pathophysiology, and therefore in its treatment, emerge.

Controversies about how to treat acne correctly still continue, and today the search for treatments, drugs, techniques, therapies, and optimal doses continues. The idea is to discover a more personalized treatment for each case. Such controversies contribute to obtaining more truths as alternatives, and, therefore, better treatments; that is, new effective drugs, but with fewer adverse effects. Yes, there is still much to learn and discover in this matter, and the technique of experimentation, can continue to offer better treatments to patients. (Ruiz, 2018).

On the other hand, the impact of acne on the quality of life of the individual who suffers from it is significant, as it directly affects their emotions and their interaction with the rest of society. In this regard, it is highlighted that approximately 2.5% of people with acne in the adolescent stage present depressive symptoms (Karnik, et al, 2014). This is because puberty is a stage where the individual tries to form his or her own identity, and seeks to fit into social groups of interest, however, suffering from acne creates shame, low self-esteem, discouragement, and anxiety; creating a barrier to social inclusion.

Considering all the above, the present work provides general aspects about acne, specifically, its etiology, pathophysiology, typologies and treatments. The study includes an explanation of the etymology or pathogenesis of the disease, marking its origin; conceptualizations about acne as a dermatological disease, from different theoretical perspectives; a description of the pathophysiology of acne focused on the different types of lesions present; typologies or classifications of acne according to its types and degrees; and an analysis of the different types of treatments used to treat acne, according to its etiology and diagnosis, such as: hormonal, topical, phototherapeutic and systemic.From the methodological perspective, the research is descriptive-documentary, based on the search of bibliographic information, mainly in books in the area of dermatology; in scientific articles published in indexed journals, about aesthetics, beauty and health; in Clinical Practice Guides; and in the International Classification of Diseases (ICD-10 and ICD-11). In addition, information was taken from the Ministry of Public Health of Ecuador; the National Directorate of Standardization; the Skin Center (CEPI), the Chilean Society of Dermatology and Venerology, the European Academy of Dermatology, the Global Alliance to Improve Acne Outcomes, the World Health Organization, the United Nations Children's Fund (UNICEF), among others, in order to obtain statistics and identify scientific evidence and recommendations.

**CHAPTER I**

**ACNE: ETIOLOGY AND DEFINITION**

This chapter shows the origin, pathogenesis or causes of acne as a dermatological disease; from the medical etiology, ancient and current. Once the etiological aspects of acne have been established, we proceed to present a series of definitions of the term, from the point of view of various researchers, and the conceptualization of acne from the author's opinion.

## Etiology or Pathogenesis of Acne

In the health sciences, to speak of "etiology" is to know the causality of a disease; it is a word used in a similar way to the term "pathogenesis", which specifically refers to the origin of a medical pathology. Therefore, under this subtopic we will talk, from different theoretical postulates, about the origin or causes of acne as a skin disease, which is essential to provide the appropriate treatment to each person who suffers from it.

The pathogenesis of acne became an interesting subject thanks to the great masters and researchers of the subject from different periods, who wrote their observations and discoveries, some of which were controversial, but which shed light on the pathogenesis of the disease. For example, Alibert credited its cause to seborrhea; Bazin and Durhing focused on the follicles and the sebaceous gland. Additionally, professors such as Shuster, Witkowski, Sulzberger Strauss, Pochi, Parish, Cunliffe, emphasized that sebaceous secretion is what causes irritation, causing follicular hyperkeratosis. (Ruiz, 2018).

Later, in 1958, Strauss and Kligman carried out an interesting work where they studied fifty biopsies of sebaceous glands, reporting their histological, chemical and physical findings of acne; reaching the conclusion that it was the sebum that could initiate the process, but it was evidenced that not all pilosebaceous units showed the same result, therefore, there was susceptibility. Such research marked the beginning of the pathology, so it was concluded that acne was a disease of the pilosebaceous follicle with increased sebum production, intraductal hyperkeratosis, proliferation of Propionibacterium acnes and inflammation, as a disturbed response of innate immunity. (Ruiz, 2018).

The most generalized idea is that acne is caused by organic factors associated with processes in the skin cells, such as: sebaceous hypersecretion, androgen stimulation, variations in the keratinocyte, Propionibacterium acnes propagation, changes in the cutaneous microbiota, increased sebum production, increased sebaceous gland size, fatty acid production, alterations in the immune system, among others. (Tanghetti, 2013; Thibouto, et al, 2009; Ottaviani, Camera, & Picardo, 2010). Regarding the increase in sebum production, it is worth clarifying that, in patients with acne, it originates due to the increase in blood levels of androgens or also due to an excessive response of the sebaceous glands to androgens.

From the point of view of Gálvez & Herrera (2006), there are several factors involved in the etiopathogenesis of acne, which have become the main objective of its treatment, namely:

•       Alteration in follicular keratinization. When there is production of a denser keratin there is an obstruction of the pilosebaceous follicle, which undergoes dilation, causing the formation of a comedo.

•       Sebaceous hypersecretion. It occurs with the onset of androgen-dependent sebaceous hyperactivity, producing enlargement of the sebaceous glands.

•       Bacterial proliferation. When comedones are present, an anaerobic environment with a high lipid component is created, which favors the proliferation of the Propionibacterium acnes bacteria.

- Inflammation. It is caused by bacterial colonization, as secondary to the release of chemotactic substances by the bacterium Propionibacterium acnes, neutrophils accumulate in and around the follicles, releasing hydrolytic enzymes, causing an inflammatory cascade.

In accordance with the above, Orozco, Campo, & Anaya, (2011) explain that the important factors in the pathogenesis of acne have been basically summarized in four, which have been widely accepted worldwide, these are: excessive increase in sebum production by the sebaceous glands; abnormal alterations in the keratinization process; presence, colonization and proliferation of the follicular bacterium Propionibacterium acnes; and constant release of inflammatory mediators in the skin.

With this in mind, the original step in the pathogenesis of acne is the so-called follicular plugging manifested as a comedo, which is produced by an uncommon desquamation of the keratinocyte in the follicular ostium. This obstruction gives way to the proliferation of Propionibacterium acnes. None of the above could occur were it not for adrenarche, which marks the onset of puberty and causes increased sebum production. At a later stage, androgens will contribute to maintain this phenomenon and also cause an increase in the size of the sebaceous gland (Gollnick & Cunliffe, 2003; Zaenglein & Thiboutot, 2006; Harper, 2004).

During this process, the composition of sebum changes, producing a large amount of free fatty acids which, together with keratin, give rise to an inflammatory process that manifests externally in the skin; and it is by the action of bacterial lipases that diglycerides, monoglycerides and free fatty acids are formed within the sebaceous follicle (Gollnick & Cunliffe, 2003; Zaenglein & Thiboutot, 2006; Harper, 2004). It should be noted that these inflammatory processes occur early in the progression of acne lesions, and the usual expression and secretion of interleukin-1 (IL-1) in non-inflamed skin increases significantly at the onset of acne development (Tanghetti, 2013).

On the other hand, as for Propionibacterium Acnes, it will induce the production of antimicrobial peptides, inflammatory cytokines, and

metalloproteinases from activated cells (Beylot, et al, 2014; Nagy, et al, 2005); and thus the formation of comedones (Beylot, et al, 2014). It is sebum that provides the substrate for the growth of Propionibacterium Acnes (McGinl, Webster, Ruggieri, & Leyden, 1978). It has been demonstrated over time that, although the amount of Propionibacterium acnes is very similar in the flora of healthy individuals and individuals with acne, the strains present in individuals with the declared disease, present genetically determined virulence factors that are not observed in strains associated with healthy individuals (Fitz-Gibbon, et al, 2013). In other words, strains differ in their inflammatory potential, which may influence the severity of acne lesions (Jasson, et al, 2013).

In addition to the above, Fierro-Arias, (2019) explains that acne as an inflammatory dermatosis that affects the pilosebaceous unit, is considered a multifactorial process, where different components are involved, such as: hormonal, infectious, hereditary, immunological, cosmetic, psychological, emotional, psychosocial, environmental, nutritional, among others. Therefore, its study must contemplate a series of physiopathogenic elements, in order to particularize the therapeutic strategies and treatments to be used.

On the other hand, Bernabeu, (2008) basically highlights three factors that cause acne lesions:

x *Hyperseborrhea*, i.e. increased sebum production by the sebaceous gland due to hormonal action. This happens mainly in adolescence, where testosterone levels increase. Through the action of the enzyme 5-alpha-reductase, testosterone is converted into dihydrotestosterone (DHT), which leads to increased sebum production.

x *Hyperkeratinization*, or the formation of microcomedones caused by abnormal proliferation of sebaceous gland keratinocytes.

x *Bacterial proliferation*, which is caused by excess sebum and hyperkeratinization, creating an anaerobic environment that induces bacterial proliferation of some bacteria of the normal skin flora, such as Corinebacterium acnes and Propionibacterium acnes. These bacteria release lipases and proteases which hydrolyze sebum triglycerides producing free fatty acids, which are irritating and comedogenic. These acids in turn attract neutrophils and macrophages leading to the appearance of inflammatory lesions.

Bernabeu (2008) adds that the appearance of acne is also associated with genetic, hereditary, psychological and emotional factors, the use of medications, the application of certain cosmetics, and hormonal factors such as those produced during pregnancy or menstruation.

As can be observed, most authors presenting the etiology or pathogenesis of acne agree that there are several factors involved in its origin, mainly those associated with processes in the skin cells, such as: sebaceous hypersecretion, intraductal hyperkeratosis, variations in the keratinocyte, abnormal stimulation of androgens, propagation of Propionibacterium acnes, production of antimicrobial peptides, changes in the cutaneous microbiota, hyperseborrhea, enlargement of the sebaceous gland, production of fatty acids, inflammatory processes, alterations in the immune system, among others. However, (Fierro-Arias, 2019; Bernabeu, 2008), add other factors that, thanks to studies carried out, have evidenced the appearance of acne; among which are:

hormonal, infectious, hereditary, immunological, cosmetic, psychological, mood, psychosocial, environmental, nutritional, medicinal, among others. In another order of ideas, throughout history a series of myths have arisen about the appearance, origin, causes and treatments of acne. The following chart shows a contrast between the most common myths and realities about acne:

*Table 1. Myths and Facts about Acne*

| Myths | Realities |
|---|---|
| Chocolate and dairy products cause acne | Studies have been conducted on this subject, however, there is no significant evidence that proves a direct relationship between the intake of dairy chocolate and the appearance of acne. |
| Stress exacerbates or causes acne | Stress causes an increase in the secretion of adrenal steroids and androgens, and therefore sebum, which exacerbates acne. That is why stress is listed among the pathogenic factors of acne. |
| Frequent washing of the face during the day decreases the production of pimples or blackheads. | Excessive facial cleansing is unfavorable for the skin, as it can eliminate its protective barrier and favor the entry of microorganisms and cause sensitization to topical treatments. |
| Acne disappears with the sun's rays | There are limited studies with significant evidence showing the efficacy of the sun against acne lesions. In addition, during acne treatment, there are antibiotics that can act as toxic agents in sunlight. |
| Acne improves with sexual intercourse | This is a completely false statement. There is no relation between acne conditions and sexual relations. |
| Acne lesions can be covered with cosmetics | There is no significant evidence that the use of cosmetics exacerbates acne, however, the use of cosmetic products to prevent acne is not indicated. If make-up is to be used during an acneic process, it is recommended to use oil-free products; non-comedogenic, i.e., that do not induce the appearance of open and closed comedones, and non-photosensitizing, i.e., that do not produce future allergies. |

*Source: Ministry of Public Health (2015), based on Australas J Dermatol 1974; Myths in Acne 2009; Acne and stress. 2007; Perceptions of acne vulgaris in final year medical student written examination answers. 2001.*

*Table No. 1* clearly shows that the pathogenesis of acne associated with the consumption of chocolates and dairy products is not proven, since there is no significant evidence that demonstrates a direct relationship between the intake of these foods and the appearance of acne; the same is true for the use of cosmetics; there is insufficient evidence to show that the use of cosmetics exacerbates acne.On the contrary, as for the hypothesis on whether stress produces acne or not, it has been proven that this emotional condition produces an increase in the secretion of adrenal steroids and androgens, and therefore of sebum, which exacerbates acne. This is the reason why stress is listed among the pathogenic factors of acne. In a later chapter we will go deeper into the treatments that have been scientifically proven to help reduce the effects of acne and even cure it. This will help to clarify some of the myths presented in *Table No. 1* about whether frequent washing of the face during the day makes the production of pimples or blackheads decrease; whether the sun's rays make acne disappear; whether sexual relations contribute to acne improvement; among other myths.

## Acne from different theoretical perspectives

According to the Medciclopedia Illustrated Dictionary of Medical Terms (2018), acne is the dermatologic condition caused by abnormal desquamation of the follicular epithelium that causes obstruction of the pilosebaceous canal with the corresponding formation of comedones. For its part, the Dictionary of the Royal Spanish Academy defines it as a skin disease characterized by chronic inflammation of the sebaceous glands, especially on the face and back. (Real Academia Española, 2019).

On the other hand, Arnal, (n/d) associates the term acne with folliculitis, that is, infection of the hair follicles, where acne originates. These follicles are a kind of sheaths where hairs are born, which have attached sebaceous glands, producing sebum or grease. When the secretion of the sebaceous glands is retained, as it is not eliminated naturally by the skin, due to its excess, its functioning is altered, causing skin inflammations and infections.

Taking these definitions as a reference, acne is a skin disorder that occurs when hair follicles become clogged with dead cells and accumulated oil, causing inflammation. It usually causes the appearance of comedones, blackheads or pimples, and is usually reflected on the face, forehead, chest, upper back and shoulders. Although it affects people of all ages, it is more frequent and common in adolescents.

Acne can also manifest itself with non-inflammatory lesions, which occur when the epidermis is altered, forming comedones with whiteheads or blackheads. However, when the lesion is inflammatory, it is due to the action of bacteria, mainly Propionibacterium acnes, which triggers inflammatory effects that can cause the rupture of the sebaceous gland and dermal inflammations of different intensity. (Ochando & Pèdèflous, 2007; Piquero, Herane, Naccha, & Molina, 2007).

In this same sense, Batlle (n/d) explains that acne is one of the most frequent and common dermatological diseases, characterized by severe inflammation of the sebaceous glands, mainly on the face, back and arms. It is not in itself a serious disease, however, it greatly affects the quality of life of those who suffer from it. Grimalt (n/d) also mentions that it is a multifactorial disorder of the pilosebaceous unit, present with manifestations caused by multiple factors, and that it affects the pilosebaceous unit due to Propionibacterium acnes and other types of bacteria.

There is no full knowledge of the ultimate trigger that causes all the manifestations of acne, however, there are a number of factors that can influence the sebaceous gland, which is a fundamental participant in the dermatological disease. Some of these factors include: increased sebum production, follicular obstruction, keratinization of the follicular duct, microbial development, lipolysis due to the action of microbial flora (Propionibacterium acnes), alteration of sexual hormones, among others.

This last mentioned factor is a good cause of the disease, since the androgenic stimulation in puberty is responsible for inciting the development of the sebaceous glands; therefore, acne would be the consequence of an imbalance of androgens and estrogens in the patient. (Cunliffe, 1989).

In summary, acne is a dermatological or skin disease, with a high impact on society, that starts when the skin pores become clogged with dead skin cells, or with the oil produced by the sebaceous glands. This happens because the production of extra sebum can clog the skin pores, causing the growth of a bacterium called Propionibacterium acnes or more commonly known as P. acnes. The process is accentuated when white blood cells attack the aforementioned bacteria, generating mild, moderate or severe inflammation of the skin. Acne varies depending on its degree of manifestation, and its causative factors are basically genetics, nutrition, hormonal changes, infections, hygiene, and stress.


## A particular conception of Acne


Acne is a variable and complex skin disease caused by the obstruction and subsequent infection and inflammation of the sebaceous duct. It begins when the skin pores become clogged with dead skin cells, or with oil produced by the sebaceous glands. This happens because the production of extra sebum can clog the skin pores, causing the growth of a bacterium called Propionibacterium acnes or more commonly known as P. acnes. The process is accentuated when white blood cells attack the aforementioned bacteria, generating mild, moderate or severe skin inflammation.

It has been scientifically proven that this dermatological disease, although not life-threatening, does deteriorate the quality of life. It can have a great physical, social and psychological impact on those who suffer from it, since it deteriorates their quality of life, as a result of emotional instability. The psychological and social disorders that occur in patients with acne produce low self-esteem, self-doubt, depression, shame, frustration, anger, confusion, poor body image, problems in the family nucleus, difficulties in work dynamics, social isolation, among other things.

In people with active acne, it is common for dysmorphophobia to be present, a disease characterized by an exaggerated concern for the presence of unwanted physical characteristics, specifically, for skin conditions that distort a person's image. Some people create in their mind the so-called "imaginary ugliness" and may spend hours in front of a mirror, turning the image perceived by them into a real obsession. All this leads to clinical depression, social phobia or obsessive compulsive disorder. Hence the importance of treating acne properly.

**CHAPTER II**

**ACNE: PATHOPHYSIOLOGY**

This chapter studies the pathophysiology or functional changes associated with acne. To speak of pathophysiology is to refer to the study of both physical and chemical pathological processes that take place in living organisms during the execution of their functions. It studies all those mechanisms of disease creation at the molecular, subcellular, cellular, tissue, organic and anatomical levels. Thus, this section will address the chemical and physical processes at the organic, anatomical, molecular and cellular levels that occur in individuals who develop acne.

## Acne and its Pathophysiology

As already mentioned in the section on acne etiology, there are primary pathogenic factors for the appearance of acne lesions, which are basically summarized in five: stimulation of the sebaceous gland; epidermal dysfunction, alteration of the keratinization process; anaerobic environment and dermal reaction, due to the presence of bacteria and sebum; follicular colonization by the bacterium Propionibacterium acnes, release of inflammatory mediators; and dysfunction of the sebaceous gland, consolidation of sebum, formation of cysts. (Nast, Dreno, Bettoli, & Degitz, 2012; Palacios, 2008).

Calzada (2009) explains that acne involves four primary pathogenic factors that interact with each other to generate lesions: sebum production by the sebaceous glands; follicular colonization by *Propionibacterium acnes*; alteration in the follicular keratinization process; and the release of inflammatory mediators into the skin. There are many types of acne lesions, which can be visualized in Table 2; and their classically accepted evolution has been that microcomedones represent predecessor lesions of acne that can evolve into non-inflammatory or inflammatory lesions.

Nast, et al (2012), Palacios (2008) and Calzada (2009) agree that the appearance of acne is the result of primary pathogenic factors, which are basically oriented towards alterations of the sebum-producing glands and the keratization process. They agree that a key factor for its complication is the follicular colonization of the Propionibacterium acnes bacteria, as well as the release of inflammatory mediators to the skin. It is important to note that Calzada (2009) does not specifically mention sebaceous gland dysfunction as a pathogenic factor, however, he refers to it when he talks about the abnormal production of sebum by the glands and the obstruction of its outflow duct.

From another perspective, Sanagustín (2017), explains that pathophysiologically two phases of acne can be distinguished: the non-inflammatory phase and the inflammatory phase. The first is characterized by increased sebum production and hyperkeratinization, leading to comedones, which can be blackheads or whiteheads; the latter can lead to the second phase: the inflammatory phase, which is due to the release of inflammatory mediators and the reproduction of the Propionibacterium acnes bacterium from whiteheads. In this phase papules, pustules, nodules, cysts and abscesses appear.

In summary, Grimalt, (n/d) explains that the initial lesion or microcomedone, represents the result of the obstruction of the sebaceous follicles by excess oil or sebum, together with desquamated epithelial cells coming from the follicular wall, which is known as ductal hyperkeratosis. Both factors cause non-inflammatory lesions such as open comedones, called blackheads or blackheads, and microcysts or closed comedones, also known as whiteheads. Later, with the proliferation of P. acnes bacteria, inflammatory mediators appear, causing superficial and deep lesions.

*Table 2. Elementary lesions in acne*

| Types of Injuries | | Graphical Representation |
|---|---|---|
| Non-inflammatory | Comedones or blackheads<br><br>xBlack (open) points<br><br>xWhite points (closed) | Comedón Cerrado — Comedón Abierto |
| Inflammatory | Superficial<br>xErythematous papules<br>xPustules<br><br>Deep<br>xNodules<br>xCysts<br>xAbscesses | Pápulas — Pústulas<br>Quistes — Nódulos<br>Abscesos |
| Scars | Derived from excess collagen<br>xHypertrophic scars<br>xQueloids<br><br>Collagen derivatives<br>xPunctate scars<br>xDeep        fibrotic scars<br>xSoft scars<br>xAtrophy<br><br>Post-inflammatory pigmentations | Cicatrices |

*Source: Own elaboration based on* (Calzada, 2009).
*Images: Own elaboration based on fragments of photographs taken from Google Images.*

As can be observed, *Table No. 2* shows the three types of elementary acne lesions: non-inflammatory, inflammatory and scarring. With regard to non-inflammatory ones, as mentioned by Sanagustín (2017), it gives rise to comedones or blackheads, known as blackheads and whiteheads, as a consequence of sebum production and hyperkeratinization. On the other hand, inflammatory lesions give rise to papules, pustules, nodules, cysts and abscesses, which, according to Calzada (2009), are classified as superficial (papules and pustules) and deep (nodules, cysts and abscesses).

Regarding scars, Calzada (2009) presents three types, those derived from collagen excess, among which are hypertrophic and keloids; those derived from collagen defect, such as: punctiform scars, deep fibrotic scars; soft scars, and atrophy; and finally, post-inflammatory pigmentation type scars. Scarring in the skin is the repair of a continuity solution by the formation of connective tissue. To understand this a little better, it is important to know the meaning of each of the types of scars, which can be visualized in *Table No. 3*, constructed from Nast, et al (2012) and Arenas (2009):

*Table 3. Types of Scars*

| Ranking | Sub-classification | Definition |
| --- | --- | --- |
| Atrophic scars | | They are very common scars, divided into three types |
| | *Scars in a box* | They are round or oval scars, with vertical edges, tend to be on the surface. slightly wider. Appearance: "U" shape |
| | *Ice pick scars* | They are deep, narrow, punctiform scars. The opening is typically wider than its depth. Appearance: Shape of "V" |
| | *Roll scars* | They are wider scars. The dermis is "glued" to the subcutaneous cellular tissue, Appearance: "M" shape. |
| Hypertrophic scar | | They are typically pink, raised, firm scars with thick collagen fibers. hyalinized, takes place within the borders of the original acne lesion site. |
| Keloid scars | | They are scars that give rise to neoformations of nodular or papular appearance, reddish-violet in color, which proliferate beyond the edges of the original wound. This type of scars occur predominantly in the trunk. |

*Source: Own elaboration, based on Nast, et al (2012) and Arenas (2009).*

In this regard, it can be added that scars are sequelae left by acne and can cause depression, decreased quality of life, and psychosocial disorders. So far there is no single technique to cure the physical scars left by acne, however, a combination of pharmacological treatments and procedures adapted to each need, can report good results over time.

Finally, among other pathogenic factors of acne, unrelated to the organic components and functions of the skin, the following can be found: genetics, racial factors, physiological factors such as the menstrual cycle and pregnancy, eating habits, climate, stress, use of cosmetics, use of certain medications such as corticosteroids, tricyclic antidepressants, diphenylhydantoins, lithium, vitamin B derivatives, among others, which could influence the appearance of acne.

# CHAPTER III

## ACNE: TYPOLOGIES

This chapter studies the different types of acne based on several theoretical postulates. To speak of typologies is to know the types or models used to classify something. Typology is considered a science that studies the classes or types of a matter in question; or the conceptual and intuitive difference of things. It is commonly used in terms of systematic studies in different areas with the purpose of defining categories. In this particular case, it is intended to classify acne by focusing specifically on its various manifestations, symptoms and degrees.

## Classification of Acne

The classification of acne has always been a controversial issue, however, for the purposes of this research, acne typologies based on the International Classification of Diseases - ICD, a key instrument for the identification of trends and statistics in the health sector worldwide, will be considered. It is made up of approximately 55,000 unique codes for injuries, diseases and causes of death. Its importance lies in providing a common language that facilitates the transmission of health information worldwide. (World Health Organization, 2018). ICD-10, classifies acne as follows:

Table 4. International Classification of Acne (ICD-10)

| Type of Acne | Definition |
| --- | --- |
| Acne vulgaris | A common form of acne that predominantly affects adolescents and young adults. Acne vulgaris probably derives from the effect of androgenic hormones and Propionibacterium acnes on the hair follicle. |
| Acne conglobate | Severe form of acne with formation of abscesses, cysts, scars and keloids. Acne conglobata may settle in the lower back, buttocks and thighs, as well as on the face and thorax. Also called cystic acne |
| Varioliform acne | A rather rare form of acne, located on the forehead. Pustules occur in two groups, each with a hard central cap. that when separating leaves a deep depression |
| Tropical acne | Form of acne caused or aggravated by high temperature and humidity. It is characterized by the presence of large nodules or pustules on the neck, back, upper arms and buttocks. |
| Infantile acne | Form of acne present between 3 and 6 months of age, but has been reported up to 16 months. Both comedonal and inflammatory acne with papules, pustules and nodules may be seen; scarring may occur. |
| Excoriated acne in young women | Form of acne that occurs in young women, with a continuous and compulsive scratching, with crushing and manipulation of pimples, blackheads and blemishes, sometimes even of normal skin. |
| Keloid acne | A form of acne with chronic irritating skin eruption of the nape of the neck, which begins as folliculitis and evolves through the formation of papules to form keloid plaques. |

Source: Ministry of Public Health (2015), based on information from WHO.

Now, according to the World Health Organization (2018), ICD-11, which represents a revision of ICD-10, will come into force from January 01, 2022. It contains a simplification of the coding structure and electronic tools. So far, ICD-11 provides for the classification of acne as follows:

*Table 5. International Classification of Acne (ICD-11)*

| Type of Acne | Definition |
|---|---|
| Comedonian acne | Acne whose main manifestation is the presence of open comedones (blackheads) or closed comedones (whiteheads). |
| Comedonian and superficial mixed acne papulopustular | Acne with comedones accompanied by small inflammatory papules and pustules. |
| Papulopustular acne | Acne whose main manifestation is the presence of multiple small inflammatory papules and pustules. |
| Nodular acne | Acne with large inflammatory nodules and fluid-filled pseudocystic lesions as well as more superficial lesions. Usually requires systemic treatment with antibiotics or retinoids. |
| Severe inflammatory acne | Intensely inflammatory acne that may be acute (acne fulminans) or subacute and chronic (acne conglobata). |
| xFulminating acne | Severe systemic disease characterized by acute inflammatory acne with multiple follicular abscesses and ulceration of the skin, accompanied by fever, thinning and arthralgias. Usually affects males.<br>white adolescents. |
| Acne conglobata | Rare chronic form of severe inflammatory acne characterized by multiple abscesses and fistulas followed by extensive hypertrophic and atrophic scarring. It may be associated with spondyloarthropathy or other follicular occlusive diseases such as dissecting cellulitis of the<br>scalp and hidradenitis suppurativa. |
| Infant acne | A form of acne that usually presents at 3-6 months of age, but later cases have been reported up to 16 months. It affects boys more often than girls, and there may be a history of severe acne in one or both parents. It may last up to 5<br>years of age. Both comedones and inflammatory acne with papules, pustules and nodules may be seen; it may leave scars. |
| Neonatal acne | Acne that manifests at birth or shortly after birth, usually with a predominance of comedones on the cheeks and few inflammatory lesions. It is thought to be due to hyperactivity of the sebaceous glands stimulated by the neonatal androgens of the<br>testicles in boys and adrenal glands in girls. |
| Acne Infantile | Infantile acne usually occurs between 3 and 6 months of age, but has been reported as early as 16 months. Male infants are affected more often than females and there may be a history of severe acne in one or more parents. It may last up to five years of age. Both comedonal and inflammatory acne with papules, pustules, and nodules may be seen; there may be scars. |
| Acne Scars | Scarring resulting from acne, ranging from a slight irregularity of the skin surface to a highly disfiguring distortion or functionally disabling of normal skin anatomy. |
| Acneiform reactions to halogenated aromatic hydrocarbons | Acne caused by exposure to halogenated hydrocarbons such as chlorinated naphthalene, dioxins and dibenzofurans. Numerous non-inflammatory comedones and cysts are a common feature. The course is usually chronic. Parts of the body frequently affected are the face, neck, armpits and groin area. |

*Source: World Health Organization (2018)*

On the other hand, there are other ways of classifying acne, among which the one established by the Ibero-Latin American College of Dermatology (CILAD), the Ibero-Latin American Group (2012), and

UNICEF (2011) can be particularly highlighted:

*Table 6. Other forms of Acne Classification*

| Categories | Type of Acne | Definition |
|---|---|---|
| **According to age** | Neonatal Acne | Form of acne presented from birth to 30 days of age. |
| | Infant acne | Form of acne presented from one month to 24 months. |
| | Acne Infantile | Form of acne presented from 2 to 10 years of age. |
| | Adolescent Acne | Form of acne presented from 10 to 19 years of age. |
| | Young Adult Acne | Form of acne presented from 20 to 24 years of age. |
| | Adult acne | Form of acne presented from the age of 25 years and older. |
| **According to grade** | Comedogenic | Acne whose main manifestation is the presence of open comedones (blackheads) or closed comedones (blackheads). white). |
| | Papulo-pustular | moderate inflammatory form of acne in which papules and pustules predominate. It may be associated with other manifestations of acne. such as comedones, nodules, and cysts |
| | Cystic nodule | severe form of acne in which nodules and cysts predominate. It may be associated with other manifestations of acne such as comedones, papules and pustules |
| **Other special shapes** | Conglobata | is a severe form manifested by multifollicular, cystic inflammatory lesions containing purulent material, forming fistulae, resistant to to treatment and producing disfiguring scars; it is predominantly located in the trunk, upper extremities and buttocks |
| | Fulminans | severe form of acne, with acute onset, characterized by systemic symptoms (malaise, fatigue, fever and arthralgias). He presents with severe inflammation of the skin, with cysts, suppuration, leukocytosis and elevated erythrocyte sedimentation rate. |

*Source: Own elaboration based on Colegio Ibero-Latinoamericano de Dermatología (CILAD), Grupo Ibero-Latinoamericano (2012) and UNICEF (2011).*

Likewise, the Illustrated Dictionary of Medical Terms Medciclopedia (2018), presents a Classification that shows some terms coincident to those already analyzed by the previously presented organisms:

*Table 7. Classification of Acne from a Medical Dictionary*

| Type of Acne | Definition |
| --- | --- |
| Acne Adenoidea | It is a type of disseminated follicular lupus. |
| Acne Agminata | A type of acne whose lesions appear in clusters. They are usually produced by the use of brominated preparations that lead to the appearance of pus-covered pustules. It is also called Barthélemy's disease. |
| Artificial Acne | It is a skin rash caused by external irritants, such as tar; or by ingesting halogenated compound. |
| Atrophic Acne | This is a type of acne in which, once the lesions disappear in the form of papules, small, reddish-greenish-black spots remain on the skin. spots, atrophic lesions and scars. |
| Cachectic Acne | It is a rash or skin irritation that usually appears in weak people, and is characterized by the formation of lesions. soft, pustular and slightly infiltrated. |
| Acne Chloride | It is a type of skin disorder showing blackish follicular papules and nails on exposed surfaces, particularly on the face, arms and neck of workers who are in contact with chlorinated compounds, such as cutting oils, varnishes, paints and lacquers. |
| Acne Conglobata | It is one of the most severe forms of acne, with the presence of abscesses, cysts, scars and keloids. This type of acne can manifest itself chronically on the face, thorax, and lower part of the face. back, buttocks and thighs. Some know it as cystic acne. |
| Acne Scoriada | It is a type of superficial acne that occurs in adolescents and young women. It is caused by compulsive squeezing of the skin. lesions already existing or about to appear, leaving scars. |
| Summer Acne | It is a type of acne characterized by keratotic papules, produced in summer or after sun exposure. It is also known as Mallorca. |
| Fulminant Acne | It is another severe form of acne, with a cystic appearance, characterized by inflamed plaques and nodules that may cause ulcers and intense scarring. The disease may manifest itself with other symptoms such as fever, arthritis, and disorders of the skin. mainly affecting adolescents. |
| Acne Indurada | It is a type of acne characterized by the appearance of large papular lesions, which almost always leave significant scarring. |
| Acne Necrotica Miliaria | It is a chronic and rare type of folliculitis of the scalp that causes the appearance of tiny pustules. It is also known as as folliculitis "Proprionibacterium acnes". |
| Acne Papulosa | It is a type of acne accompanied by small papules that do not inflammatory. It is commonly considered a papular form of acne vulgaris. |
| Acne Pustulosa | It is that form of acne in which the predominant lesions are pustular and scarring. |
| Keloid Acne | It is a chronic irritating cutaneous eruption of the nape of the neck, which starts as a kind of folliculitis, and gradually evolves forming first papules and then keloid plaques. |

| Acne Keratosis | This is a form of acne in which a horny plug takes the place of the comedo. |
|---|---|
| Acne Rosacea | It is a chronic inflammatory disease characterized by dysfunction of the sebaceous glands of the face, neck and shoulders. It produces negative ocular effects such as blepharoconjunctivitis. chronic, catarrhal marginal ulcers, episcleritis and iritis. |
| Tropical Acne | It is a type of acne caused by high temperatures and high humidity. It shows the presence of large nodules or pustules on the skin. neck, upper arms, back and buttocks. |
| Acne Urticarialis | It is the form of acne characterized by edematous papules in the shape of haloes, which are aggravated by scratching. |
| Varioliform acne | It is a rare type of acne that manifests on the forehead. It is characterized by the formation of pustules, which occur in two groups, each with a hard central plug that when separated leaves a deep depression. |
| Acne Vulgaris | It is the usual and most common form of acne, affecting mainly adolescents and young adults. It is probably produced by the effect of androgenic hormones and the Propionibacterium acnes on the hair follicle. |

Source: Medciclopedia (2018)

Finally, acne can also be classified according to the degree of severity, into mild, moderate and severe acne. Mild acne presents non-inflammatory lesions in the form of comedones, as well as scarce papulo-pustular inflammatory lesions; moderate acne is characterized by superficial inflammatory lesions and occasional nodules; and severe acne manifests extensive inflammatory lesions, nodules and scars. Moderate acne becomes severe when, after six months of treatment, no improvement is observed, in addition to the fact of presenting acute psychological conditions in those who suffer from it. (Purdy & Berker, 2011) In summary, it can be said that there is a great variety of forms of presentation of acne. Not all authors, ministries, organizations and health institutions mentioned in this research classify it in the same way, but they all agree that, depending on age, sex, degree, level of inflammation, types of lesions present, symptomatology, pathophysiology, among other things, it should be assigned a different name, so that the health professional knows what pathology is present, in order to administer the most appropriate treatment.

# CHAPTER IV

## ACNE: TREATMENTS

The consequences of acne on the patient will depend on a good treatment, which will influence the quality of life during the disease and in the future. This chapter presents the different types of treatments that can be administered to a patient to cure, stop or improve acne. Treatments considered are: Hormonal, Topical, Phototherapeutic and Systemic. This section aims to explain in which cases a treatment is appropriate and in which cases it is not; when to use a certain treatment; how to combine them when necessary; dosages, duration time, among other things.

## How to treat acne

Acne is a disease and must be accepted and treated as such. In recent years there have been important therapeutic advances in the field of acne. However, according to Muñoz (2001), the success in the effectiveness of acne treatment depends a lot on the patient and his family environment, as well as the origin and correct diagnosis given by the specialist, considering the intensity in which the pathology is presented, the clinical form of acne and the associated etiological factors of each individual suffering from the disease.

There are a variety of ways to treat acne, ranging from home methods, herbal methods, to systemic and professional methods, with the application of medications prescribed by dermatological specialists. When choosing a treatment, it is important to take into account that each skin type is different, and that each origin is particular, therefore, the effects may vary from person to person, so it is not to be expected exactly the same results in everyone who suffers from acne.

Acne treatment basically focuses on correcting the etiological factors that stimulate its appearance, i.e. reducing bacteria, regulating sebaceous secretion, preventing obstruction of the hair follicle, avoiding the formation of comedones, among others. The clinical spectrum varies greatly, as there may be a discreet facial comedonal acne, or a very severe nodulocystic acne of the face, neck and back. Therefore, treatments vary, they can be hormonal, phototherapeutic, topical, systemic or surgical, and the ideal treatment must be chosen for each type of patient.

In addition to the pathogenesis of acne, the appropriate treatment of acne depends on the knowledge of three important aspects: severity, intensity and level of functional alteration. Firstly, severity is determined by its extension, which indicates the number of areas involved, as well as the percentage of involvement. Secondly, the intensity depends on the type of lesion and the presence of comedones, papules, pustules, nodules, cysts and scars left by the disease. Finally, the degree of functional alteration is measured by the emotional commitment of each patient suffering from the disease, the level of disturbance it has generated in their quality of life, and other psychological factors such as anxiety and depression.

The choice of the appropriate treatment will depend on several factors, such as the clinical form of the disease or pathophysiology, the severity and the patient's response to previous treatments. If the disease is mild, it can be treated in a single phase, but if it is chronic, the treatment should be based on two stages, an initial phase to achieve an effective reduction in the depth and extent of the lesions, and a second maintenance phase focused on the prevention of relapses or exacerbations of acne. Additionally, the result of the treatment will depend on the compliance that each patient gives to it, so an adequate doctor-patient relationship will be essential. (Orozco, Campo, Anaya, et al, 2011) When starting treatment, it is essential that the treating physician makes the patient aware that the therapy will last for a long time, making it clear that the improvement will probably not be immediate, and that there may even be a worsening at the beginning. In order to encourage compliance with the treatment, the physician should keep the patient constantly informed, since the dermatologist usually prescribes different active ingredients simultaneously and changes them according to the evolution of the disease, and the patient should be aware of this. It is also important to emphasize that until at least three months after the beginning of the treatment, a reasonable judgment of its efficacy cannot be made, therefore, the patient should not be discouraged.The following is an explanation of the different types of treatments that can be used to treat acne pathologies. *Figure No. 1* shows the classification of therapies that, according to the author's criteria, should be used to treat the aforementioned disease.

*Figure 1. Acne Treatments according to Pathogenesis*

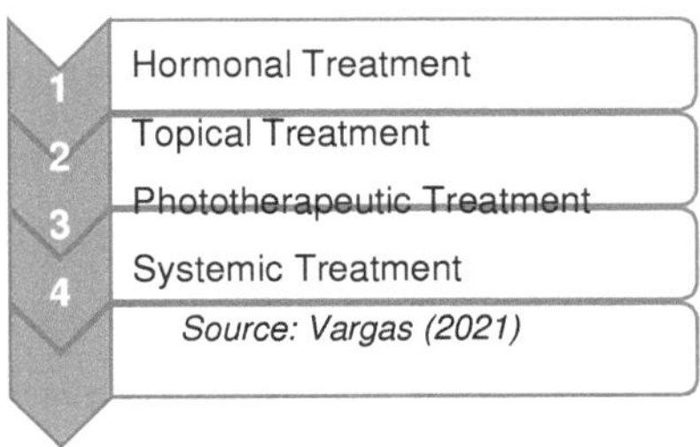

## Hormonal Treatment

Androgens, i.e. male sex hormones corresponding to testosterone, androsterone and androstenedione, secreted by the testicles in men and by the ovaries in women, play a very important role in the pathogenesis of acne, and in the absence of these hormones the pathology does not develop. Hormonal treatment is seen by many as an alternative to systemic acne treatment or as an adjunct to it. Hormonal treatment can be used in women diagnosed with severe seborrhea, androgenic alopecia, seborrhea-alopecia-hirsutism-acne syndrome - SAHA, premenstrual flare-ups or late-onset acne (Koo, Petersen, & Kimball, 2014; Tyler & Zirwas, 2013; Dalamaga, et al, 2013).

The most recent advances in the etiology of acne have shown that sebaceous hyperproduction and follicular keratinization, two of the four main factors in the pathogenesis of acne, are triggered by the action of androgens, i.e. hormones that stimulate the development of sexual characteristics, mostly secreted by the testicles in men and also by the ovaries in women. This has led to the development of new acne treatment strategies based on hormonal therapies, known as HT.

For example, some women have found the use of contraceptives to treat acne to be successful, resulting in an improvement in their episodes of menstrual acne. The reason for this is that the birth control pill produces a protein called sex hormone binding globulin (SHBG), which absorbs testosterone, thereby increasing the relative levels of estrogen in the blood. When there is an increase in androgen levels, oral therapy is essential, which is why oral contraceptives with anti-androgen effect are used, as well as cyproterone acetate and flutamide. In addition, isotretinoin at low doses is very useful as therapy alone or in conjunction with contraceptives. There are two large groups of hormonal treatments for acne: non-contraceptive HTs that include agents such as: spironolactone, cyproterone acetate and flutamide; and hormonal contraceptives (HA), consisting of an estrogenic and a progestin component. With regard to HA combinations to treat acne, the U.S. Food and Drug Administration has approved the following: ethinylestradiol 20/30/35 mg + norethindrone 1 mg; ethinylestradiol 35 mg + norgestimate 180/215/250 mg; and ethinylestradiol 20 mg + drosperinone 3 mg. On the other hand, in Canada the following combinations can also be used: ethinylestradiol 35 mg + cyproterone acetate 2 mg, ethinylestradiol 35 mg + levonorgestrel 100 mg and ethinylestradiol 35 mg + drosperinone 3 mg. (Husein- ElAhmed & Ortega-Del Olmo, 2013).In summary, there are many therapeutic treatments with anti-androgenic action that block, so to speak, the effect of male hormones on the skin and scalp. Among the most commonly used are: cyproterone acetate, flutamide, spironolactone and drospirenone, as well as isotretinoin alone or together with contraceptives. Regarding hormonal contraceptives, the most commonly used are: ethinylestradiol, norethindrone, norgestimate, drosperinone, levonorgestrel and drosperinone. The contraceptives recommended as acne treatment act by reducing follicular hyperkeratinization and decreasing sebum production in the sebaceous glands, thus improving the appearance of the skin and preventing the appearance of new acne lesions.

*Table 8. Hormonal treatments for acne*

| Type of Treatment | Medication Recommended | Approved Combinations to treat acne |
|---|---|---|
| HT Non Contraceptive | Spironolactone | x Ethinylestradiol 20/30/35 mg + Norethindrone 1 mg |
| | Cyproterone Acetate | x Ethinylestradiol 35 mg + Norgestimate 180/215/250 mg |
| | Flutamide | |
| | Isotretinoin | x Ethinylestradiol 20 mg + Drosperinone 3 mg |
| | Ethinyl estradiol | |

| TH Contraceptives | Norethindrone | x Ethinylestradiol 35 mg + Cyproterone Acetate 2 mg |
|---|---|---|
| | Norgestimate | x Ethinylestradiol 35 mg + Levonorgestrel 100 mg |
| | Drosperinone | x Ethinylestradiol 35 mg + Drosperinone 3 mg |
| | Levonorgestrel | |
| | Drosperinone | |

*Source: Own elaboration, based on Husein-ElAhmed & Ortega-Del Olmo, (2013) and U.S. Food and Drug Administration.*

## Topical Treatment

Topical treatments are indicated mainly in patients with non-inflammatory acne lesions, mild inflammatory acne, moderate inflammatory acne, or comedonal acne (Gollnick, et al, 2003). These types of acne often do not require specialized medical attention; they can be treated by cosmiatrists, dermocosmiatrists and cosmetologists; or, in some cases in conjunction with a dermatologist, since the combination of systemic and topical treatments to treat acne lesions is totally valid.

Depending on the pathogenesis, there are a variety of topical options to treat acne. The most common are: the use of topical antibiotics such as erythromycin, dapsone and clindamycin; benzoyl peroxide, sulfur, sodium sulfacetamide, azelaic acid, salicylic acid and retinoids. Specifically for the treatment of comedonal and inflammatory acne, retinoids and benzoyl peroxide are recommended (Rathi, 2011; Cunliffe, 1998).

Additionally, there are also other treatment modalities such as superficial chemical dermabrasion, a technique that, through the use of topical chemicals, it is possible to produce an abrasion on the skin to improve its quality. (Keri & Shiman, 2009). However, in cases with high inflammation and many lesions, a medical specialist may prescribe oral medication to the patient, combined with topical treatments.

Acid-based chemical peels are also widely used. One of the most commonly used for the regulation of oil production is glycolic acid in concentrations of 10 to 20%, especially in patients with acne where comedones are still present and scars predominate. However, it is important to clarify that the use of chemical exfoliators in concentrations of 35 to 50% for more intense dermabrasion is the responsibility of a dermatologist. These chemical substances based on glycolic acid have an advantage, they are not photosensitizing, that is, they do not cause side effects on the skin when in contact with light, so they do not produce a noticeable desquamation on the patient's skin. (Peñaloza, 2003).

*Table 9. Most common topical treatments used on acne lesions*

| Type of Treatment Topic | Treatment | Features and Functions | Recommendations in its administration |
|---|---|---|---|
| **Antibioti** | Clindamycin Dapsone and Erythromycin | Decrease the bacterial population P. acnes They have properties anti-inflammatory The association of erythromycin with benzoyl peroxide allows for the reduction of of the risk of bacterial resistance | Clindamycin should administered at 1% and the erythromycin at 2% or 4%. The addition of zinc to erythromycin and clindamycin enhances its efficacy therapeutics Erythromycin should not be used never alone Clindamycin alone is better than the erythromycin. The major effect of the clindamycin is obtained from after 6 weeks of use The risk of resistance to erythromycin may be reduced by using a erythromycin-containing gel at 3% and benzoyl peroxide at 5%. |

| **cs Topics** | | | It is recommended to combine<br>1% clindamycin and 1% clindamycin peroxide.<br>5% benzoyl.<br>Efficacy of antibiotics topics increases with the addition of benzoyl peroxide or a retinoid<br>It is recommended to administer topical antibiotics between 8 and 12 weeks continuous. |
| | Sodium sulfacetamide | Recommended for inflammatory processes associated with bacterial infection and in combination with sulfur has properties<br><br>antibacterial, antifungals, antidemodex and effect keratolytic | Can be used in combination with with sulfur from the following way: Sodium sulfacetamide 10% + 5% sulfur |

| | | | |
|---|---|---|---|
| **Topical antibacterials** | Benzoyl peroxide | Improves inflammatory and non-inflammatory lesions. Reduces the percentage of free fatty acids. Eliminates acne-causing bacteria Eliminates dead skin cells that clog pores Inhibits the appearance of antibiotic-resistant strains. | For the moderate type of acne can be used only It is formulated in cream, gel, lotion and soap, in concentrations of 2.5, the 5, 7.5 and 10%. Must be applied with care as it may discolor hair and clothing. |
| | Retinoid Topical isotretinoin (13-cisretinoic acid) | It is anti-inflammatory and comedolytic It does not inhibit sebum formation and is not bactericidal, it is associated with an antibacterial agent. It is less irritating than tretinoin. It is photosensitizing. | Use at 0.05% in gel |

| | Retinoid Tretinoin (all-transretinoic acid) | Normalize desquamation of the follicular epithelium. Promotes the drainage of pre-existing comedones Inhibits the formation of comedones of new comedones Reduces the growth of Propionibacterium acnes Power penetration of other drugs Diminishes hypertrophic scars left by acne | Apply only at night Should be applied with dry skin to avoid further desquamative process. |
|---|---|---|---|
| | Retinoid Adapalene | Has comedolytic and anti-inflammatory activity Reduces open and closed comedones and is very active on inflammatory lesions | It is applied at 0.1% in gel or cream 0.1% adapalene and 2.5% benzoyl peroxide are useful in patients with higher lesion counts May produce erythema, dryness, moderate itching and pruritus. It can be used during the summer, as it has not been used during the summer. observed cases of photosensitivity Should be avoided during pregnancy |
| | Retinoid Tazarotene | It acts on epidermal hyperproliferation and on the gamma nuclear receptors | Mild to moderate irritation No is photosensitizing. |

| | | | |
|---|---|---|---|
| **Other topical alternatives** | Sulfur | It has an important germicidal, fungicidal, parasiticide and keratolytic action. Removes dead skin cells that clog pores Helps remove excess oil | Apply only on the affected areas Use with caution in areas of acute inflammation. Should not be applied near the eyes Do not use on blistered, burned or wounded areas. If irritation is observed, discontinue use immediately. Can be combined with sulfacetamide, salicylic acid, benzoyl peroxide and resorcinol. Sulfur tends to leave the skin dry, so it is recommended that you use gradualization in the time of permanence of the product on skin, and moisturizing with products fat-free |
| | Alpha Hydroxy Acids (Glycolic Acid and Lactic Acid) | They help eliminate dead skin cells and reduce inflammation caused by acne. Stimulates the growth of new, smoother skin. Improves the appearance of acne scars Makes pores look smoother. perceived to be smaller. | They can cause irritation, to avoid this it is suggested to start with a small amount and gradually increase it. |
| | Azelaic Acid | It acts against blackheads and swelling caused by acne | Do not use more than the indicated dose or more often than prescribed by the physician. physician |

| Salicylic Acid | Eliminates and prevents the appearance of blackheads. Reduce swelling and redness Opens clogged skin pores, allowing pimples to dry out. Helps prevent blackheads from clog pores | It is recommended to prepare a sufficient quantity to cover the affected area; dilute the powder to form a smooth paste. May cause skin irritation |
| --- | --- | --- |



As can be seen in the table above, an important topical option to treat acne is the combination of topical antibiotics with other organic and chemical compounds, such as benzoyl peroxide or retinoids. The association of a topical retinoid with benzoyl peroxide is another important option, however, it can produce irritation in the patient. In the latter situation, the retinoid should be applied at night and the benzoyl peroxide in the morning. In addition, it is important to note that the association of a topical retinoid with a topical antibiotic is a good option to consider, however, antibiotic resistance may initiate a problem in the patient. (Guerra, et al, 2015).

In this order of ideas, Gollnick, et al (2003) point out that for the topical treatment of acne, fixed combinations of active ingredients are indicated in patients presenting non-inflammatory lesions, or mild or moderate inflammatory acne. Furthermore, according to Lookingbill, et al (1997) and Guerra (2012), scientific clinical studies have shown that fixed combinations are a fundamental therapeutic guideline for acne, because of their high efficacy and low level of side effects.

*Table 10. Tested topical treatment associations*

| Association | Result |
| --- | --- |
| Benzoyl peroxide + Retinoid (Adapalene) | Activation of Antimicrobial Activity + Decreased of microcomedone formation |
| Benzoyl peroxide + Antibiotic (Clindamycin) | Antimicrobial Activity Activation + Suspension of bacterial multiplication |
| Antibiotic (Clindamycin) + Retinoid (Adapalene) | Suspension of the multiplication of bacteria + Reduction of the number and size of comedones |
| Isotretinoin + Erythromycin | Decreased sebum and growth reduction of Propionibacterium acnes + Decrease of infection |
| Tretinoin + Erythromycin | Reduction of the hyperkeratinization process that leads to the formation of microcomedones + Decrease in the number of microcomedones + Decrease in the number of microcomedones + Decrease in the number of microcomedones of infection |

*Source: Own elaboration, based on Orozco, et al (2011); Torras & Mascaró (2007).*

It is clear then, that in topical therapy for acne, single substances can be used or associated with antibiotics; it is also possible to combine topical treatments with systemic treatments. The table above shows associations of topical treatments proven to treat acne. Combinations of Antibiotics with Antibacterials such as Benzoyl Peroxide, Antibiotics with Retinoids, Antibiotics with Vitamins, but also combinations of organic and chemical substances such as Retinoids with Antibacterials such as Benzoyl Peroxide can be seen. According to the European Academy of Dermatology, topical retinoids have a medium level of recommendation for the treatment of comedonal and papulopustular acne, but a high level combined with Benzoyl Peroxide.

# Phototherapeutic Treatment

Phototherapeutic treatments for acne are generally indicated when a topical treatment is insufficient. Phototherapy is a technique used through natural or artificial electromagnetic radiation for the treatment of many diseases, but it has been mainly useful in skin pathologies. The light applied can be visible, infrared or ultraviolet radiation. (Royal National Academy of Medicine, 2012). In a contrary opinion, Berneburg, et al (2008), explain that the common electromagnetic spectrum in dermatological treatments ranges from visible light to the infrared level; clarifying that the ultraviolet range is not employed, since ionizing radiation is not administered. However, for the purpose of this research, phototherapeutic treatments based on a varied electromagnetic spectrum are included.

Thanks to the emission of blue light, which penetrates into the deepest layers of the skin, the bacteria that cause acne can be removed and the regeneration of the epidermis can be excited, contributing greatly to the reduction of inflammation, disappearance of lesions, and reduction of scars or sequelae left by acne. This is why phototherapeutic treatments are fundamental in this type of dermatological pathologies, and have represented a good option when topical treatment does not give the expected results.

There are basically two types of dermatological phototherapies: laser and pulsed light (blue, red, infrared). Both differ in that laser technology emits a single wave of light, while pulsed light emits many rays of light that can cover a larger area of skin at the time of treatment. In either case there is an emission of light, which reaches the tissues producing the effects described by Anderson and Parrish in 1983, in the theory of selective photothermolysis (Trelles, Levy, & Ghersetich, 2008), which consists of the specific destruction of a cellular structure or chromophore, due to the thermal increase induced by electromagnetic radiation.

With respect to laser therapy, it is important to clarify that once light reaches the skin, it has four possible functions: to be reflected, absorbed, scattered or transmitted; but the effect on tissues can only occur when the light is absorbed (Hirsch & Anderson, 2003; Carroll & Humphreys, 2006; Austen, Goldsmith, & Fitzpatrick, 2003). Laser treatment is used primarily to eliminate the bacteria that cause acne, as well as a very thin layer of skin, which helps reduce scarring. The procedure consists of destroying the sebaceous glands that generate excess oil in the skin, in order to reduce infection and improve inflammatory acne lesions. It is effective not only in getting rid of existing pimples, but also in stopping new outbreaks.

As for pulsed light, it does not have the same capacity of the laser to be coherent and perform displacements in the same amplitude and direction; it is based on the generation of a non-coherent polychromatic light source of high intensity. According to Medina & Rodriguez (2013), pulsed light is used by applying various filters according to the problem to be treated, which help to use a specific waveform; the light is released in lapses of one, two or three pulses of two to 25 min duration on average achieving a large skin coverage during the application. This procedure reduces sebaceous secretion, i.e. excess oil production.

In order to produce the desired effect, the light should be absorbed by the target tissue to convert it into heat energy, so the biological effect is determined by the temperature reached, i.e. the longer the wavelength, the greater the penetration of the light into the tissue. It is important to clarify that not all the light that strikes the skin surface is absorbed by the target chromophore. A large amount of the light is scattered, and some is transmitted through the target chromophore, so that only a small amount is reflected. Thus, the larger the beam size, the lesser the scattering.

(Medina & Rodriguez, 2013).

On the other hand, an additional alternative is Photodynamic Therapy (PDT), used to treat a variety of dermatoesthetic conditions, including acne. This technique consists of administering a photosensitizing compound that accumulates in the target cells, and after an incubation period, illuminating with light of a wavelength within the absorption spectrum of the photosensitizer. The effect is caused by photoactivation of the sensitizer in the tissue to be treated, leading to oxidative damage of a wide variety of target cells. As a final result, the destruction of the abnormal or cancerous tissue can be obtained, which is caused by the synthesis of reactive monoatomic oxygen and the oxidative damage caused by free radicals in the altered cells and in the endothelial cells of the abnormal neovessels (Martínez & Trelles, 2010; Moreno, Alvarado, & Camps, 2007; Ruiz & Rebollo, 2009; Uebelhoer & Dover, 2005).

Another modern breakthrough in acne treatment is Biophotonic Therapy. Unlike other treatments, this therapy uses a light conversion system designed to stimulate the skin's own repair mechanisms at the cellular level. Through a multi-wavelength LED light in combination with a photoconverter gel, biophotonic technology allows a spectrum of wavelengths to penetrate the skin, stimulating collagen formation, which can aid in the repair of scars produced as a result of acne (DermoMedic, 2017).

Biophotonic Therapy is a unique light conversion technique designed to stimulate the skin's own repair mechanisms at the cellular level. This innovative acne treatment combines a lamp capable of emitting multiple wavelengths of light through LEDs with a photoconverter gel. This gel allows the spectrum of wavelengths to penetrate into the deepest layer of the skin, allowing the elimination of bacteria, decreasing sebaceous secretion and improving inflammation. Biophotonic Therapy acts against acne while stimulating collagen production, which helps eliminate acne scars.

In summary, laser, intense pulsed light (IPL), light emitting diode (LED) systems and photodynamic therapy (PDT) are major advances in dermatological medicine, techniques that are currently used to treat various skin diseases through the emission of light, which is why they are considered phototherapeutic treatments. The light produces conductive waves of energy, which cause a specific destruction of the cellular structure or chromophore; activate fibroblasts, help in the production of collagen and elastin; stimulate at the cellular level the repair mechanisms of the skin, among other positive effects.

*Table 11. Phototherapeutic treatments for acne*

| Phototherapy | Energy Type | Function |
|---|---|---|
| Laser | | Laser treatment is used to fight the bacteria that cause acne, as well as remove a very thin layer of skin, reducing the appearance of acne lesions and scars. |
| Pulsed light | Blue Light | Blue light has the ability to penetrate the skin and produce oxygen radicals that aid in the destruction of acne-causing bacteria. It also produces inflammation-reducing effects, preventing future outbreaks. |
| | Red Light | Red light promotes skin regeneration, reducing inflammation and strengthening skin elasticity. Red light waves contribute to the improvement of acne and to skin rejuvenation by activating the fibroblasts responsible for the formation of the skin. collagen and elastin. |
| | Infrared Light | Infrared uses a long wavelength, therefore, it can penetrate deep into the skin. It activates fibroblasts, which are responsible for the formation of collagen and elastin, whose fibers help to maintain the skin. It is used to treat acne lesions and improve the appearance of the skin. acne scars. |

| | Suitable laser light within the absorptio n spectrum of the photosens itizer | Photodynamic therapy consists of the administration of a photosensitizing agent on the affected tissue in combination with a specific light irradiation, causing tissue destruction. which eliminates acne-causing bacteria. |
|---|---|---|
| Photodynami c Therapy (PTD) | | |
| Biophotonic Therapy | Multi-waveleng th LED light | Biophotonic Therapy through a multi-wavelength LED light in combination with a photoconverting gel acts against acne while stimulating collagen production, which helps to eliminate acne scars. |



## Systemic Treatment

A systemic treatment is appropriate in the severe active phase of acne, and even more so when inflammatory signs are widely present. Generally, systemic treatment is used when a patient has not responded to previous treatments, or has not been successful with topical or even phototherapeutic therapies; its main objective being to act on the etiopathogenic factors involved, namely: alterations in follicular keratinization; sebaceous hypersecretion; bacterial proliferation; and inflammation.For systemic therapy, drugs classified into three major groups are used: antibiotics; hormonal; and isotretinoin. The latter, isotretinoin, continues to be the most effective treatment in the therapy of cystic nodule acne or acne with a severe scar component. It should be noted that, in more recent times, new macrolide antibiotics have been developed with similar results to tetracyclines, and new oral contraceptives with lower amounts of estrogens and new progestogens are available. Additionally, new drugs for systemic use are being developed, such as zileuton, insulin-sensitizing drugs and oligonucleotides, which have the ability to block androgen receptors of the sebaceous glands. (Gálvez & Herrera, 2006) In the same vein, Keri &

Shiman (2009) explain that to treat acne pathology, systemic treatment is very frequently used. Such therapy includes the use of systemic antibiotics, oral contraceptives, antiandrogens and retinoids. Gonzalez & Nottola (2007) refer to the following groups as alternative systemic treatments for acne: systemic antibiotics, oral contraceptives, antiandrogens and oral isotretinoin.

*Table 12. Systemic Acne Treatments*

| Groups of Drugs | Sub - Groups of Drugs | Drugs | Dose Recommended | Effect |
|---|---|---|---|---|
| Systemic Antibiotics | Tetracyclines | Doxycycline | 100 mg per day for 12 weeks | Antibacterial Anti-inflammatory |
| | | Minocycline | 100 mg per day up to 200 mg per day, for 12 months. weeks | |
| | | Limecycline | 150-300 mg per day, for 12 weeks | |
| | Macrolides | Erythromycin | 500 mg every 12 hours for about 6 weeks | |
| | | Clarithromycin | 500 mg per day | |
| | | Azithromycin | 500 mg daily for three days | |
| | | Roxithromycin | 300 mg per day | |
| | Quinolones | Ciprofloxacin | 500-750 mg each 12 hours during 7-14 days | |
| | | lomefloxacin | 400 mg per day for 10 days | |
| | | ofloxacin | 400 mg daily | |
| | | pefloxacin | 400 mg every 12 hours | |
| | Sulfamides | Dapsone | 100 mg/day for 3 months | |
| | Diaminopyr | Trimetho | 800 mg/day of |

| | | imidines | prim | 7-10 days | |
| | | Diaminopyrimidine + sulfonamides | Trimethoprim-Sulfamethoxazole | 160 mg trimethoprim and 800 mg sulfamethoxazole | |
| Systemic Hormonal Therapy | Antiandrogens | Spironolactone | 250 to 500 mg daily in two doses dosage | | Antibacterial Anti-inflammatory |
| | | Flutamide | From 62.5 to 250 mg daily in a single dose | | |
| | | Drospirenone | 30 mg / day | | |
| | | Cyproterone | 50 to 100 mg per day | | |
| | | Metformin | 500 mg increased weekly up to 2.000 mg per day | | |
| | Contraceptives | Ethinyl estradiol Norethindrone Norgestimate Drospirenone Levonorgestrel Drosperinone | 1 tablet daily, unless another dose is suggested by the treating physician | | |
| Systemic Retinoids | | Isotretinoin | 0.5 mg/kg/d up to a cumulative dose of 150 mg/kg for a period of 0.5 mg/kg/d up to a cumulative dose of 150 mg/kg for a period of 0.5 mg/kg/d. | | Keratolytic Anticomedogenic Antimicrobacterial Anti-inflammatory |

| | | | from 16 to 20 weeks | |
|---|---|---|---|---|
| | | | | |
| Other Alternativ es Systemi c | Nitroimidaz oles | Metronid azole | 7.5 mg/kg body weight every 6 days hours | Antimicrob ial |



As can be seen, all the authors mentioned in this section agree on the type of treatment that should be administered from the systemic point of view. The theory expressed shows some small discrepancies, but, in the long run, they convey the same idea. For example, Gálvez & Herrera (2006) speak of only three major groups: antibiotics; hormonal drugs; and isotretinoin; for their part, both Keri & Shiman (2009) and González & Nottola (2007), refer to four groups: systemic antibiotics, oral contraceptives, anti-androgens, and retinoids; making the remark that oral isotretinoin is a synthetic retinoid, derived from retinol, also known as 13-cis-retinoic acid, therefore, these last authors present the same classification. It is important to clarify that, although Gálvez & Herrera (2006) refer to hormonal drugs, and not to oral contraceptives; and to antiandrogens, in short, they are talking about the same thing.

## Some specific treatments according to type of acne

Up to this point, a range of treatments commonly used to treat acne pathologies have been addressed, with techniques and procedures that vary according to the type of acne, etiology, intensity, and severity, which have been used according to new discoveries in the area. The following is a series of topical, systemic and hormonal treatments compiled from the perspective of various authors, and recommended depending on the type of pathology present.

*Table 13. Some topical, systemic and hormonal treatments according to type of pathology*

| Type of Acne | Feature Pathological | Treatment |
|---|---|---|
| Acne Comedonica | Normal skin | Topical Retinoids are used, such as: tretinoin, adapalene and tazarotene, which act by modifying follicular dyskeratosis, have a keratolytic effect, that is, they produce desquamation and sometimes irritation. |
| | Thick or very oily skin | Use adapalene at a level greater than 0.1 % or tretainoin at a higher percentage of 0.1 %. 0,025%. |
| | Sensitive skin | Use adapalene 0.1% or tretainoin 0.025%. Administer on alternate days and at night, due to its photosensitizing action. |
| Acne Papulo - Pustular | Mildly present on the face | Use benzoyl peroxide, which has a keratolytic and bacteriostatic effect, so it acts both at the level of Propionibacterium acne and in follicular dyskeratosis, at 4 or 5% is well tolerated. It should be administered at night due to its photosensitizing effects. |
| | Present in the upper trunk in a mild form. | Use 10% benzoyl peroxide only at night. |
| | Comedonic component important | Combine and apply clindamycin with benzoyl peroxide, or erythromycin with tretinoin to different percentages. |
| | Moderate and Severe | A combined treatment of oral antibiotics with tetracyclines such as doxycycline and Minocycline should be performed, plus some topical protocol. The recommended dose of doxycycline and minocycline is 100 mg per day. |
| | Patients who do not respond to conventional treatment | In this case, treatment with isotretinoin should be administered. |
| Acne Cystic nodule | Moderate and Severe | It will require isotretinoin as treatment with a conventional dose of 0.5 to 1mg/kg bw/day. At the end of this treatment, topical retinoid |

|  |  | should be administered routinely for at least 2 weeks. at least 3 months. |
|---|---|---|
| Acne associated with hyperandrogeni sm | Hormonal | The use of free testosterone, Dehydroepiandrosterone Sulfate (DHEAS), androstenedione, LH, FSH, 17 Hydroxyprogesterone and prolactin |
|  | Congenital adrenal hyperplasia + acne | Treatment should be based on oral corticosteroid with minimal dosage; the following is preferred dexamethasone 0.6mg administered at night. |
|  | Hyperandrog enism of ovarian origin | Administer drugs with anti-androgenic effect, that is, a combination of estrogens with cyproterone acetate, or failing that, drosperinone or its equivalents. It should be noted that if the levels of androgens are very high, the following should be administered parallel antiandrogens, either Cyproterone or Butamide. |
|  | Elevated prolactin | Multidisciplinary treatment is administered aimed at correcting hyperprolactinemia |

*Source: Own elaboration, based on Diez (2009); Zaenglein & Thiboutot (2006); Harper (2004); Plewig & Kligman (2000); Gollnick & Cunliffe (2003); Krowchuk (2000); Skidmore, et al (2003); (Van Vloten, et al (2002); Warren (2007).*

In addition to the above, the table below provides a variety of hormonal, topical and systemic treatments to treat different types of acne, with three basic choices, and a fourth alternative where the condition is present in women with signs of androgenization. The information was taken from the Guía Práctica Clínica de Diagnóstico y tratamiento del acné (Clinical Practice Guide for the Diagnosis and Treatment of Acne), proposed by the Ministry of Public Health of Ecuador. This guide has been adapted by professionals from the institutions of the National Health System and expert specialists in acne, under the coordination of the National Directorate of Standardization of the Ecuadorian Ministry of Public Health. In it, scientific evidence and suggestions have been compiled in order to assist health professionals and patients in making a decision about the diagnosis and treatment of this pathology.

Table 14. Some Treatments of Choice

| Type of Acne | First Election | Second Election | Third Election | Women with signs of androgenization |
|---|---|---|---|---|
| **Acne**<br><br>**Slight** | Retinoid<br><br>topical +/-<br><br>antibiotic topical(PBO) | Topical retinoid alternative + other antibiotic | Topical retinoid alternative + another antibiotic | Topical retinoid + topical antibiotic (PBO) |
| **Acne**<br><br>**Moderate** | Oral antibiotic (doxycycline)+ retinoid topical +/-<br><br>PBO*<br>PBO*<br>PBO*<br>PBO*<br>PBO*<br>PBO*<br>PBO*<br>PBO*<br>PBO | Oral antibiotic alternative + topical retinoid +/-<br><br>PBO * PBO *<br>PBO * PBO *<br>PBO * PBO *<br>PBO * PBO *<br>PBO | Oral antibiotic alternative + topical retinoid anternative +<br><br>PBO * PBO * PBO *<br>PBO * PBO * PBO *<br>PBO * PBO * PBO | Contraceptives combined oral + topical retinoid +/- antibiotic topic |
| **Acne**<br><br>**Severo** | Isotretinoin oral** | High dose of oral antibiotic + topical retinoid + PBO | Dapsone oral + PBO | Antiandrogen at high dose + topical retinoid +/- topical antibiotic or isotretinoin+ contraceptives antiandrogenic drugs |
| **Special shapes:**<br><br>**Conglobat a fulminas** | Oral isotretinoin + systemic corticosteroid for the first few weeks | Dapsone + topical antibiotic + PBO | High-dose oral antibiotic + topical retinoid + PBO | See first choice of special shapes |
| **Maintenance** | | Topical retinoid | Topical retinoid + PBO | |
| **Scars**<br><br>**Hypertrophica** | Infiltration with steroids | Techniques surgical procedures. | Treatments ablatives without evidence scientific | |

| Scars | Tretinoin***. | Microdermoa brasi | Techniques |  |
|---|---|---|---|---|
| **Hypert rophic a** | 0.25% - 0.5% adapalene | s website | surgical |  |
|  |  | laser | (excision, punch |  |
|  | 0.1% | treatment with microneedles | y subdivision |  |

Source: Ministry of Public Health (2015).

Throughout this article the possible treatments that can be used to treat the pathology of acne have been explained in detail. Although there is some variability among the various guidelines for the pharmacological treatment applied to acne, in general a gradual and progressive treatment is recommended depending on the severity and the results that are visualized. In cases of mild acne, as a first option, a topical monotherapy treatment can be chosen, based on benzoyl peroxide, retinoids and azelaic acid; a second option is to combine topical treatments, i.e. antibiotics with benzoyl, antibiotics with retinoids, or antibiotics with acids; as a third option topical medications combined with systemic antibiotics are recommended; and, finally, the use of systemic retinoids is suggested, and in women, oral contraceptives.It is important to consider that, when making a decision to start a pharmacological treatment for acne, an individualized choice should be applied, depending on the pathogenesis, severity, intensity and clinical presentation, without leaving aside the psychological and social factor of the patient. Additionally, it is necessary to take into account the efficacy of the therapy applied and how it has been tolerated; the skin phototype; the potential compliance according to the location of the lesions; the difficulties presented in its application; and, of course, the cost of the treatment. As acne is a multifactorial disease, with varied clinical presentations, a combined treatment at fixed doses can be very useful.

# CONCLUSIONS

Acne is a dermatological disease that starts when the skin pores become clogged with dead skin cells, or oil produced by the sebaceous glands. This happens because the production of extra sebum can clog the skin pores, causing the growth of a bacterium called *Propionibacterium Acnes* or more commonly known as *P. acnes.*

In acne there are primary pathogenic factors that interact with each other to generate lesions, among the most important are the production of sebum by the sebaceous glands; follicular colonization by *Propionibacterium acnes*; the alteration in the process of follicular keratinization; and the release of inflammatory mediators to the skin. But there are also other pathogenic factors of acne, unrelated to the components and organic functions of the skin, such as genetics, racial factors, physiological factors such as the menstrual cycle and pregnancy, eating habits, climate, stress, use of cosmetics, use of certain medications.

The three types of elementary acne lesions are non-inflammatory, inflammatory and scarring. Non-inflammatory lesions result in comedones or blackheads, known as blackheads and whiteheads, as a consequence of sebum production and hyperkeratinization. On the other hand, inflammatory lesions give rise to papules, pustules, nodules, cysts and abscesses, which are classified as superficial (papules and pustules) and deep (nodules, cysts and abscesses).

In view of the wide range of existing typologies of acne, an important reference for cataloguing it is the International Classification of Diseases - ICD, a key instrument for the identification of trends and statistics in the health sector worldwide. Its importance lies in providing a common language that facilitates the transmission of health information worldwide. This does not mean that the rest of the classifications presented by other authors, institutions and organizations are not valid, however, the unification of health language worldwide is achieved through the ICD.

Acne is a multifactorial disease and, as such, its treatment must be professionally thought out and come from an expert specialist in the field. Self-medicating or following treatments provided by miracle cosmetics would not be the right thing to do, as this would rather contribute to improve the evolution of acne, and turn a generally mild condition into something serious or severe.

In order to treat acne, it is essential to find the causative factor, that is, to discover its pathogenesis, which allows the most appropriate and effective therapy to be recommended. The treatment that the physician recommends to a patient will depend on his or her age, origin, intensity of the condition, severity of the acne, and level of functional alteration.

There is a wide range of therapeutic actions that can be used to treat acne pathologies, among which are: hormonal, topical, phototherapeutic and systemic treatments, as well as other types of therapies that, in the opinion of the experts, are considered appropriate to apply.

The techniques used to treat this pathology range from classical compounds to very complex formulas of topical application, including hormonal and systemic procedures with the use of drugs, as well as the combination of modern methods and therapies. No treatment is better than the other; its efficacy will depend on the detection of the pathogenesis and the diagnosis made by the specialist or treating physician.Acne medications have the particularity of reducing the production of oil produced in the sebaceous glands, speeding up the renewal of dermal cells, reducing or ending bacterial infection, reducing inflammation levels, and preventing scarring.

With most medications given to treat acne, you may not see good results right away, and your skin may even get worse before it gets better. So a key aspect of the patient's recovery is to be aware that it may take months, or even years, for the acne to completely clear up.

In addition to topical and systemic treatments, in the modern era it is increasingly common to use technology, devices and devices to deliver acne therapies. Light system treatments, for example, have proven to be effective, and may be comparable to those obtained when oral antibiotics are administered; however, light system therapies result in faster resolution, with fewer side effects, and, most importantly, greater patient satisfaction for the sufferer.

After all of the above, it is concluded that, although not all authors, ministries, organizations and health institutions mentioned in this research classify acne in the same way, they do agree that, depending on age, sex, degree, level of inflammation, types of lesions present, symptomatology, pathophysiology, among other things, it should be assigned a different name, so that the health professional knows what pathology he/she is facing, in order to administer the appropriate treatment.

As a general conclusion, today we are in the presence of a compendium of multiple therapeutic possibilities to treat acne, which have not remained in simple topical protocols, systemic therapies, or hormonal treatments, but go beyond. Finally, in order to achieve the appropriate treatment, specific aspects and situations must be observed in each patient, such as the clinical type of acne, the specific diagnosis, its intensity and severity, the skin phototype, and the degree of collaboration; in order to be able to cure or control the pathology effectively.

# BIBLIOGRAPHIC REFERENCES

Abdel-Naser, M., & Zouboulis, C. (noviembre de 2008). Tretinoin gel formulation in the treatment of acne vulgaris. *Expert Opin Pharmacother, 9*(16), 2931-7. doi:10.1517/14656566.9.16.2931

Akman, A., Durusoy, C., Senturk, M., Koc, C., Soyturk, D., & Alpsoy, E. (2007). Treatment of acne with intermittent and conventional isotretinoin: a randomized, controlled multicenter study. *Archives of dermatological research, 299*(10), 467-473.

Arenas, R. (2009). *Dermatology: Atlas, diagnosis and treatment* (4th ed.). Mexico City: Mc Graw Hill.

Arnal, M.(n/d). *A word every day: Acne.*Retrievedfrom http://www.elalmanaqu.com/lexico/acne.htm

Austen, K., Goldsmith, L., S., K., & Fitzpatrick, T. (2003). *Dermatology in General Medicine*
(6 ed.). McGraw-Hill.

Batlle, C. (n/d). Acne treatment. *Dermofarmacia Magazine.*

Bernabeu, A. (2008). Acne. Etiology and treatment. *Elsevier, 27*(8), 76-80.

Berneburg, M., Trelles, M., Friguet, B., Ogden, S., Esrefoglu, M., Kaya, G., . . . Thappa, D. (2008). How best to halt and/or revert UV-induced skin ageing: Strategies, facts and fiction. *Controversies in Experimental Dermatology, 17*, 228.

Beylot, C., Auffret, N., Poli, F., Claudel, J., Leccia, M., Giudice, P., & al., e. (2014). Propionibacterium acnes: An update on its rolein the pathogenesis of acne. *J Eur Acad Dermatol Venereol*(28), 271---8.

Bhambri, S., Del Rosso, J., & Desai, A. (2007). Oral trimethoprim/sulfamethoxazole in the treatment of acne vulgaris. *CUTIS-NEW YORK, 79*(6), 430.

Brandstetter, A., & Howard, I. (2011). Topical dose justification: benzoyl peroxide concentrations. *Journal of Dermatological Treatment, 24*(4), 275-277.

Brodell, R., Schlosser, B., Rafal, E., & al., e. (2012). A fixed-dose combination of adapalene 0.1%-BPO 2.5% allows an early and sustained improvement in quality of life and patient treatment satisfaction in severe acne. *J Dermatolog Treat, 23*(1), 26-34.

Calzada, G. (Oct-Dec 2009). Pediatric dermatology: what's new in acne? *Rev Pediatr Aten Primaria , 11*(17). doi:doi:10.4321/S1139

Carroll, L., & Humphreys, T. (2006). LASER-tissue interactions. *Clin Dermatol, 24*(1), 2-7.

Ibero-Latin American College of Dermatology (CILAD) and the Ibero-Latin American Group of. (2012). Acne a Global Approach. (5), 63-69. Retrieved from http://www.cilad.org/archivos/1/GILEA/clasific2012.pdf

Cunliffe W, e. a. (1998). A comparison of the efficacy and tolerability of adapalene 0.1% gel versus tretinoin 0.025% gel in patients with acne vulgaris: a meta-analysis of five randomized trials. *The British journal of dermatology*(139), 48-56.

Cunliffe, W. (1989). Acne: sebaceous gland phisiology. *Londres: Duritx*, 123-139.

Dalamaga, M.,Papadavid,E.,Basios,G.,Vaggopoulos, V., Rigopoulos, D., Kassanos,

D.,

& & Trakakis, E. (2013). Ovarian SAHA syndrome is associated with a more insulin-resistant proile and represents an independent risk factor for glucose abnormalities in wome with polycystic ovary syndrome: A prospective controlled study. *Journal of the American Academy of Dermatology, 69*(6), 922-930.

DermoMedic. (February 8, 2017). *Biophotonic therapy for acne lesions.* Retrieved from dermomedic.com: https://dermomedic.com/terapia-biofotonica-lesiones-del-acne/

Diez, J. (2009). Rational management of acne. *Rev Soc Bol Ped , 48*(1), 24-30.

Feldman, S., Tan, J., Poulin, Y., Dirschka, T., Kerrouche, N., & Manna, V. (2011). the efficacy of adapalenebenzoyl peroxide combination increases with number of acne lesions. *Journal of the American Academy of Dermatology, 64*(6), 1085-1091.

Fierro-Arias, L. (2019). Acne in our times. *Dermatol Rev Mex, 63*, S1-S2.

Fitz-Gibbon, S., Tomida, S., Chiu, B., Nguyen, L., Du, C., Liu, M., & al., e. a. (2013). Propionibacterium acnes strain populations in the human skin microbiome associated with acne. *J Invest Dermatol*(133), 2152---60.

Gálvez, M., & Herrera, E. (2006). Systemic treatment of acne . *Piel, 21*(4), 213-217.

Ghodsi, Z., Orawa, H., & Zouboulis, C. (2009). Prevalence, severity, and severity risk factors of acne in high school pupils: a community-based study. *Journal of Investigative Dermatology, 29*(9), 2136-2141.

Gollnick, H., & Cunliffe, W. (2003). management of acne. Areport from a global alliance to Improve Outcomes inacne. *J Am Acad Dermatol*(49), 1-38.

González, F., & Nottola, N. (2007). Treatment of polycystic ovary syndrome dermatological management. *Venezuelan Journal of Endocrinology and Metabolism, 5*(3).

Goulden, V., Stables, G., & Cunliffe, W. (1999). Prevalence of facial acne in adults . *J Am Acad Dermatol, 41*(4), 577-580.

Grimalt, S. (n/d). Acne.

Guerra, A. (2012). Effects of benzoyl peroxide 5%/clindamycin combination gel versus adapalene 0.1% on quality of life in patients with mild to moderate acne vulgaris: a randomized single-blind study. *J Drugs Dermatol*, 466-474.

Guerra, T., & al, e. (2015). Consensus on the topical treatment of acne. *Med Cutan*

*Iber Lat Am, 43*(2), 104-121.

Gupta, A. K., & al, e. ( de 2003). A randomized, double-blind, multicenter, parallel group study to compare relative efficacies of the topical gels 3% erythromycin/5% benzoyl peroxide and 0.025% tretinoin/ erythromycin 4% in the treatment of moderate acne vulgaris. *J Cutan Med Surg, 7*(1), 31-7. doi: 10.1007/s10227-002-2101-2

Harper, J. (2004). An update on the pathogenesis and management of acne vulgaris. *J Am Acad Dermatol*(51), 37-9.

Hirsch, R., & Anderson, R. (2003). Principles of laser-skin interactions. En *Bolognia JL, Jorizzo JL, Rapini R, Horn TD, Mascaro JM, Mancini AJ, Salasche SJ, Saurat JH, Stingl G, editors. Dermatology* (págs. 2143-2151). Spain.

Husein-ElAhmed, H., & Ortega-Del Olmo, R. (2013). Hormonal treatment of acne. *Skin.*
*Continuing Education in Dermatology, 28*(5), 309 - 312.

Israni, D., Mehta, T., Shah, S., & Goyal, R. (2013). Effect Of Metformin Therapy In Female Visiting Dermatologist For Acne Vulgaris Having Endocrine And Sonographic Characteristics Of Polycystic Ovary Syndrome (Pcos). *Asian Journal of Pharmaceutical and Clinical Research, 6*(2), 76-82.

Jasson, F., Nagy, I., Knol, A., Zuliani, T., Khammari, A., & Dreno, B. (2013). Different strains of Propionibacterium acnes modulate differently the cutaneous innate immunity. *Exp Dermatol*(22), 587---92.

Karnik, J., Baumann, L., Bruce, S., Callender, V., Cohen, S., Grimes, P., & Smith, S. (2014). A double-blind, randomized, multicenter, controlled trial of suspended olymethylmethacrylate microspheres for the correction of atrophic facial acne scars. *Journal of the American Academy.*

Keri, J., & Shiman, M. (2009). An update on the management of acne vulgaris . *Clin Cosmet Investig Dermatol, 2*, 105-110.

Koo, E., Petersen, D., & Kimball, B. (2014). Meta-analysis comparing eficacy of antibiotics versus oral contraceptives in acne vulgaris. *Journal of the American Academy of Dermatology.*

Krowchuk, D. (2000). Treating acne: a practical guide. *Med Clin North Am.* (84), 811–828.

Lee, J., Yoo, K., Park, K., & al., e. (2011). Effectiveness of conventional, low-dose and intermittent oral isotretinoin in the treatment of acne: a randomized, controlled comparative study. *Br J Dermatol, 164*(6), 1369-1375.

Leyden, J., Shalita, A., & Hordinsky, M. (2002). Eficacy of a low-dose oral contraceptive containing 20 g of ethinyl estradiol and 100 g of levonorgestrel for the treatment of moderate acne: A randomized, placebo-controlled trial. *47*(3), 399–409.

Lookingbill, D., Chalker, D., Lindholm, J., Katz, H., Kempers, S., Huerter, C., & al, e.

(1997). Treatment of acne with a combination clindamycin/benzoyl peroxide gel compared with clindamycin gel, benzoyl peroxide gel and vehicle gel: combined results of two double-blind investigations. *J Am Acad Dermatol*, 590-595.

Martínez, P., & Trelles, M. (2010). The role of epidermal growth factor receptor in photodynamic therapy: a review of the literature and proposal for future investigation. *Lasers Med Sci, 25*(767).

McGinl, K., Webster, G., Ruggieri, M., & Leyden, J. ( 1978). Regional vanauons m dens1ty of cutaneous propionibacteria: correlation of P. A enes populations with sebaceous secretion. *Journal of Clinical Microbiology*, 672-675.

Medciclopedia (Ed.). (2018). *Illustrated dictionary of medical terms.* Retrieved from https://www.iqb.es/diccio/a/ac2.htm

Medina, G., & Rodríguez, U. (2013). Intense pulsed light in the treatment of acne. *Rev Hosp Jua Mex, 80*(2), 129-133.

Ministry of Public Health. (2015). *Diagnosis and treatment of acne: Clinical Practice Guide. First Edition Quito: ; 2015. Available at: http://salud.gob.ec.* Ministry of Public Health, National Directorate of Standardization. Quito: Primera. Retrieved from http://salud.gob.ec

Moreno, G., A., E., Alvarado, A., & Camps, A. (2007). M Photodynamic therapy. *Med Cutan Iber Lat Am, 35*(255).

Muñoz, M. (2001). Acne and its treatment. *Offarm, 20*(8), 71-81.

Nagy, I., Pivarcsi, A., Koreck, A., Szell, M., Urban, E., & Kemeny, L. (2005). Distinct strains of Propionibacterium acnes induce selective human beta-defensin-2 and interleukin-8 expression in human keratinocytes throughtoll-like receptors. *J Invest Dermatol*(124), 931---8.

Nast, A., Dreno, B., Bettoli, V., & Degitz, K. (2012). European evidence-based (S3) guidelines for the treatment of acne. *J Eur Acad Dermatol Venereol, 26*(1), 1-29.

Ochando, M., & Pèdèflous, M. (2007). Update in the Global Treatment of Acne Vulgaris.

World Health Organization. (June 18, 2018). The World Health Organization today publishes its new international classification of diseases (ICD-11). *WHO.* Retrieved from https://www. who.int/en/news/item/17-06-2018-who-releases- new-international-classification-of-diseases-(icd-11)

Orozco, B., Campo, M., Anaya, L., & al, e. (2011). Colombian guidelines for the management of acne: an evidence-based review by the Colombian Acne Study Group. *Rev Asoc Colomb Dermatol*, 129-157.

Ottaviani, M., Camera, E., & Picardo, M. (August 25, 2010). Lipid mediators in acne. Mediators Inflamm. doi:doi: 10.1155 / 2010/858176.

Palacios, S. (2008). *Undergraduate Notebooks Morphofunction of the skin.* Pontificia Universidad Católica del Ecuador, School of Medicine.

Peñaloza, J. (August 2003). Acne. *Rev Fac Med UNAM, 46*(4).

Piquero, M., Herane, M., Naccha, E., & M., M. (2007). Pathophysiology and pathogenesis in: Acne a Global approach. *The Ibero-Latin American College of Dermatology (CILAD) and the Latin American Group for the Study of Acne (GLEA), 2,* 17-32.

Plewig, G., & Kligman, A. (2000). *Acne and rosacea* (Third ed.). New York: Springer-Verlag.

Poulin, Y., & al, e. (01 de abril de 2011). A 6-month maintenance therapy with adapalene- benzoyl peroxide gel prevents relapse and continuously improves efficacy among patients with severe acne vulgaris: results of a randomized controlled trial. *British Journal of Dermatology, 164,* 1376-1382. Obtenido de https://doi.org/10.1111/j.1365- 2133.2011.10344.x

Purdy, S., & Berker, D. (2011). Acne vulgaris. Clinical evidence. *BMJ Publishing Group,* 1714.

Rathi, S. (2011). Acne vulgaris treatment: the current scenario. *Indian J Dermatol, 56*(1), 7- 13.

Royal Spanish Academy. (2019). *Dictionary of the Spanish language.* (A. d. española, Ed.) Spain.

Royal National Medicine. (2012).*Dictionary of medical terms.* Panamericana.

Ross, J., Snelling, A., Eady, E., Cove, J., Cunliffe, W., Leyden, J., & Oshima, S. (febrero de 2001). Phenotypic and genotypic characterization of antibiotic-resistant Propionibacterium acnes isolated from acne patients attending dermatology clinics in Europe, the USA, Japan and Australia. *Br J Dermatol, 144*(2), 339-46. doi:10.1046/j.1365-2133.2001.03956.x

Ruiz, J. (2018). Acne: history and controversies. *Dermatol Rev Mex, 62*(3), 189-191.

Ruiz, J., & Rebollo, N. (2009). Photodynamic therapy in dermatology. *Dermatology Rev Mex, 53*(178).

Sanagustín, A. (March 2017). *Acne: pathophysiology and treatment.* ( Medicine and Health Blog) Retrieved October 21, 2020, from albertosanagustin: https://www.albertosanagustin.com/

Skidmore, R., Kovach, R., Walker, C., Thomas, J., Bradshaw, M., & Leyden, J. (2003). Effects of subantimicrobialdose doxycycline in the treatment of moderate acne. . *Arch Dermatol* (139), 459-464.

Strauss, J., Leyden, J., Lucky, A., Lookingbill, D., Drake, L., Haniin, J., & Hong, J. (2001). A randomized trial of the eficacy of a new micronized formulation versus a standard formulation of isotretinoin in patients with severe recalcitrant nodular acne. *Journal of the American Academy of Dermatology, 45*(2), 187-195.

Tanghetti, E. (2013). The role of inflammation in the pathology of acne. *Clin Aesthet*

*Dermatol*(6), 27-35.

Thibouto, t. D., Gollnick, H., Bettoli, V., Dreno, B., Kang, S., Leyden, J., & al., e. (2009). New insights into the management of acne: An updatefrom the Global Alliance to Improve Outcomes in Acne group. *J Am Acad Dermatol*(60), 1-50.

Torras, H., & Mascaró, J. (2007). Treatment of acne. *Piel, 22*(10), 528-534.

Trelles, M., Levy, J., & Ghersetich, I. (2008). Effects achieved on stretch marks by a non- fractional broadband infrared light system treatment. *Aesth Plastic Surg.* doi:10.1007/Soo268-008- 9115-0

Tyler, K., & Zirwas, J. (2013). Contraception and the dermatologist. *Journal of the American Academy of Dermatology, 68*(6), 1022-1029.

Uebelhoer, N., & Dover, J. (2005). Photodynamic therapy for cosmetic applications . *Dermatologic therapy , 18*(242).

UNICEF. (2011). Adolescence an age of opportunity. (UNICEF, Ed.) *The State of the World's Children 2011.*

Van Vloten, W., Haselen, C., Van Zuren, E., Gerlinger, C., & Heithecker, R. (2002). The effect of two combined oral contraceptives containing either drosperinone or cyproterone acetate on acne and seborrhea. *Cutis*(69), 2-15.

Warren, H. (2007). Oral contraceptives for the treatment of acne vulgaris. *J Am Acad Dermatol* (56), 1056-1057.

White, G. (1998). Recent findings in the epidemiologic evidence, classification, and subtypes of acne vulgaris. *J Am Acad Dermatol, 39*(2), S34-S37.

Zaenglein, A., & Thiboutot, D. (2006). Expert committee recommendations for acne management. (118), 1188-99.

Zouboulis, C., & Piquero-Martin, J. (2003). Update and future of systemic acne treatment.
*Dermatology, 206*(1), 37-53.